MW01488156

Chair Yoga For Seniors

Learn How Chair Yoga Can Help You Feel Younger and More Energetic

Dr. Ashley J. Smith

Table of Contents

Introduction

Chair Yoga For Seniors is a type of yoga that aims to keep seniors active, improve their balance and flexibility, and make them feel younger and more energetic. This style of yoga incorporates classic yoga positions as well as seated and standing postures tailored to the needs of seniors.

Chair Yoga For Seniors is an excellent approach to reap the physical and emotional benefits of yoga without requiring much space or equipment. Chair Yoga is a moderate form of exercise that requires the use of a chair for support, making it ideal for seniors who are unable to perform regular yoga poses.

Seniors can reap the benefits of greater physical activity without risk of harm by practicing Chair Yoga.

Chapter 1. Definition of Chair Yoga

Chair yoga is a wonderful activity for seniors that can help them maintain both their physical and emotional health. It is a style of yoga that caters primarily to senior citizens and other people who may have difficulty moving about. It is a kind of exercise that is low-impact and soft, and it may be done while seated in the convenience of a chair.

Chair yoga incorporates a series of poses and motions that are intended to stretch and strengthen the body, as well as increase flexibility and coordination. The benefits of chair yoga include a reduction in stress and weariness, improved cardiovascular health, and improved balance and stability.

You don't need to be particularly flexible or young to practice chair yoga; in fact, you can even perform it in the convenience of your own living room. It is a fantastic method to stay active and maintain a healthy lifestyle, and one can do it either in a group setting or on their own.

The benefits of chair yoga include an improvement in posture as well as a reduction in pain and stiffness. In addition to these benefits, it can be a helpful method for achieving relaxation and relieving stress, helping to increase mental clarity and attention.

For older citizens, chair yoga can be a wonderful way to keep connected with their peers, and it can also assist to build a sense of well-being and belonging for the participant. It is a pastime that can be enjoyed in the company of family and friends, and it may be a wonderful way to keep oneself physically and intellectually fit.

Chapter 2. Benefits of Chair Yoga for Seniors

People's bodies change as they get older, which might make it more challenging for them to participate in physically demanding activities. This might result in feelings of loneliness as well as decreased levels of energy.

Because of this, chair yoga is an excellent way for elderly people to remain active without having to be concerned about their physical limitations.

Seniors can develop their flexibility and mobility, their posture and balance, their strength, and their sense of equilibrium through the practice of chair yoga, which has many benefits. In addition to helping relieve tension and anxiety, chair yoga can also improve overall health and well-being.

Chair yoga is a wonderful kind of exercise for older people because it can be done in a setting that is both safe and comfortable. The usage of a chair offers support and stability, hence lowering the risk of harm that can be caused by falling or by other types of accidents.

Because chair yoga is easy on the joints and muscles, older citizens don't need to worry about experiencing any kind of pain or discomfort while they do it.

Chair yoga has been shown to be beneficial not just to a person's physical health but also to their mental well-being. In addition to relieving tension and anxiety, doing yoga in a chair can enhance mental clarity and attention, as well as lessen feelings of isolation.

It may also help improve your mood and sense of well-being, both of which are essential for maintaining good physical health as you get older.

By engaging multiple regions of the brain, chair yoga can even help slow down cognitive loss and dementia linked with aging. This benefit is especially beneficial for seniors. In addition, frequent chair yoga practice helps boost confidence as you become older and improves your social life by providing opportunities to engage in conversation with others who share your interest in leading healthy lifestyles.

Chapter 3. Basics of Chair Yoga

The practice of yoga that is done while seated in a chair is referred to as "chair yoga." It is frequently practiced by older people who may not be able to perform the more strenuous positions that are typically associated with conventional yoga.

The practice of yoga in a chair offers individuals the opportunity to gain many of the same advantages as traditional yoga, but with less of a burden on their bodies.

The following is some basic details regarding chair yoga for seniors that you should be aware of:

A. Equipment needed

1. Chair: A sturdy, comfortable chair that is stable and easy to move.

2. Straps: Yoga straps or large scarves to help seniors reach their full range of motion.

3. Yoga Blocks: Yoga blocks or books to help seniors maintain balance and stability.

4. Towel: A thick towel or blanket to provide cushioning and support for seniors' joints.

5. Yoga Mat: An optional yoga mat for additional cushioning and stability.

6. Music: Optional background music to help create a calming atmosphere.

7. Water: A glass of water to stay hydrated during the session.

B. Types of chairs used

The chairs that are used in chair yoga for seniors are a great tool that may be used to promote physical, mental, and emotional well-being.

Seniors can benefit from increased flexibility, strength, balance, and coordination via the practice of chair yoga, which also makes yoga more approachable. In addition to this, it provides a method that is both risk-free and comfortable for lowering levels of tension and anxiety, and it may even assist enhance overall brain clarity. Seniors can benefit greatly from staying active and interested in their personal health and fitness by participating in chair yoga.

Because it provides them with something to grab onto and assists them in maintaining their balance and stability, the use of a chair makes it simpler for seniors to do yoga poses. In addition to this benefit, it helps to lessen the risk of injuries and falls that can be caused by standing positions. In addition to that, the chair.

1. Balance Ball Chairs: These special chairs feature a large, inflatable ball that is designed to support and engage the core while allowing seniors to perform a variety of seated yoga poses.

2. Reclining Chairs: These chairs are designed to provide extra back and neck support, as well as to allow for a greater range of motion.

3. Folding Chairs: These lightweight, compact chairs are great for seniors who need more stability and support while performing chair yoga poses.

4. Meditation Chairs: These chairs are designed to provide a comfortable, upright seating position for seniors while they practice meditation and relaxation techniques.

5. Rocking Chairs: These chairs provide gentle motion and comfort while allowing seniors to perform yoga poses in a seated position.

C. Preparing the space

1. Clear any furniture or other items out of the way to create a comfortable and safe space for the yoga session.

2. Make sure the space is well-ventilated with open windows or a fan.

3. Place a yoga mat or towel in the room.

4. Place a chair in each corner of the room, ensuring that the chairs are stable and secure.

5. Place a few cushions or blankets on the chairs for extra comfort.

6. Place a water bottle and a hand towel on each chair.

7. Play soothing music to create a relaxing atmosphere.

8. Make sure the temperature is comfortable.

9. If needed, provide props such as straps, blocks, and bolsters to help the seniors with their poses.

Chapter 4. Warm-up Exercises

Warm-up exercises are essential before a senior begins chair yoga. They help to prepare the body for the upcoming yoga session by increasing the heart rate, loosening the joints and muscles, and improving circulation. Warm-up exercises also help to reduce the risk of injury and increase flexibility

. By doing warm-up exercises, seniors can gradually increase their range of motion and gradually increase the intensity of the yoga session.

Additionally, warm-up exercises can help reduce stress and improve seniors' overall wellbeing, as the exercises can be calming and grounding. Warm-up exercises also help to get seniors into the right mental and physical state for their yoga session, improving focus and concentration.

Finally, warm-up exercises can provide a great opportunity for seniors to connect with their breath and relax their minds. All these benefits of warm-up exercises make them essential before engaging in chair yoga.

Some of the warm up exercises are;

1. Neck Rolls: Begin by sitting up straight in the chair. Gently roll the head in a circular motion, moving the chin towards the right shoulder and then down towards the chest. Reverse the motion, bringing the chin up towards the left shoulder and then back to the center. Repeat this motion 3-5 times.

2. Shoulder Rolls: Sit up straight and clasp the hands together behind the back. Take a deep breath in and, as you exhale, roll the shoulders up towards the ears. Reverse the motion, bringing the shoulders back down and around. Repeat this motion 3-5 times.

3. Arm Circles: Begin by sitting up straight in the chair. Extend both arms out to the sides and make small circles in the air with the hands. Reverse the motion and repeat the circles in the opposite direction. Do this 3-5 times.

4. Chest Expansion: Sit up straight, take a deep breath in and expand the chest. As you exhale, release the chest back to the starting position. Repeat this motion 3-5 times.

5. Torso Twist: Begin by sitting up straight in the chair. Place both hands on the right knee and twist the torso to the right. Hold the position for a few seconds before releasing back to center. Repeat the motion on the left side. Do this 3-5 times.

6. Hip Flexion: Sitting up straight, extend the right leg and flex the right foot. Hold the position for a few seconds and then return the foot to the starting position. Repeat the motion on the left side. Do this 3-5 times.

7. Ankle Circles: Begin by sitting up straight in the chair. Extend the right leg and make small circles in the air with the right foot. Reverse the motion and repeat the circles in the opposite direction. Do this 3-5 times for each leg.

8. Hand Claps: Sitting up straight in the chair, clap the hands together in front of the body. Do this 3-5 times.

9. Knee Bends: Sitting up straight, extend the right leg and slightly bend the knee. Hold the position for a few seconds, and then return the foot to the starting position. Repeat the motion on the left side. Do this 3-5 times.

10. Calf Raises: Begin by sitting up straight in the chair. Extend the right leg and raise the calf off the floor. Hold the position for a few seconds and then return the foot to the starting position. Repeat the motion on the left side. Do this 3-5 times.

Chapter 5. Chair Yoga Poses

1. Seated Mountain Pose: Begin by sitting in a chair with your feet flat on the floor and your hands resting on your knees. Lift your chest and keep your spine tall, like a mountain. Hold this pose for 5-10 breaths.

Illustration:

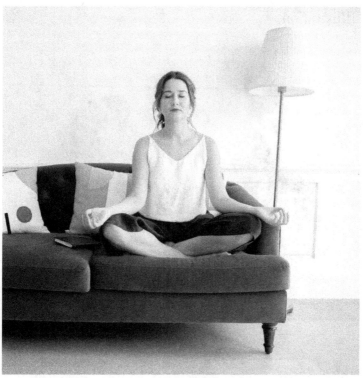

2. Seated Cat-Cow Pose: Starting in the Seated Mountain Pose, inhale and arch your back, stretching your chest forward. On the exhale, round your back, tucking your chin towards your chest. Alternate between arching and rounding your back for 5-10 breaths.

Illustration:

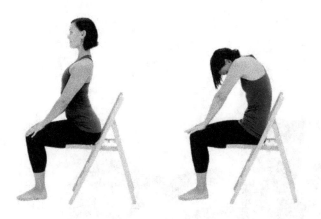

3. Seated Neck Rolls: Begin in the Seated Mountain Pose. Inhale and slowly drop your right ear to your right shoulder. Exhale and roll your head back to center. Inhale and drop your left ear to your left shoulder. Exhale and roll your head back. Repeat for 5-10 reps.

Illustration:

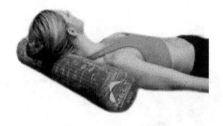

4. Seated Spinal Twist: Starting in Seated Mountain Pose, inhale and reach your right arm to the back of the chair. Exhale and twist your torso to the right. Place your left hand on the right arm of the chair for support. Hold for 5-10 breaths before returning to center and repeating on the left side.

Illustration:

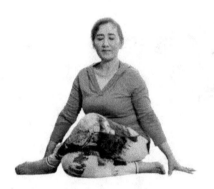

5. Seated Forward Bend: Begin in the Seated Mountain Pose. Inhale and reach your arms up to the sky. Exhale and fold forward at your hips, bringing your hands to the arms of the chair. Relax your neck and shoulders and stay here for 5-10 breaths.

Illustration:

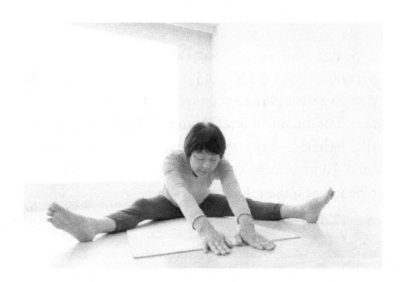

6. Seated Half Sun Salutation: Starting in the Seated Mountain Pose, inhale and reach your arms up to the sky. Exhale and fold forward at your hips, bringing your hands to the arms of the chair. Inhale and come back to Seated Mountain Pose. Exhale and reach your arms up to the sky. Repeat for 5-10 reps.

7. Seated Half Moon Pose: Begin in the Seated Mountain Pose. Inhale and reach your arms up to the sky. Exhale and reach your right arm to the back of the chair. Inhale and reach your left arm up to the sky. Exhale and twist your torso to the right. Hold for 5-10 breaths before returning to center and repeating on the left side.

8. Seated Side Bend: Begin in the Seated Mountain Pose. Inhale and reach your arms up to the sky. Exhale and reach your right arm up and to the right, stretching your left side. Hold for 5-10 breaths

before returning to center and repeating on the left side.

9. Seated Bird of Paradise Pose: Begin in the Seated Mountain Pose. Inhale and reach your arms up to the sky. Exhale and reach your right arm to the back of the chair. Inhale and reach your left arm around the outside of your right arm. Hold for 5-10 breaths before returning to center and repeating on the left side.

10. Seated Arm Circles: Begin in the Seated Mountain Pose. Inhale and reach your arms up to the sky. Exhale and circle your arms forward for 5-10 reps. Inhale and circle your arms back for 5-10 reps.

11. Seated Shoulder Shrugs: Begin in the Seated Mountain Pose. Inhale and raise your shoulders up

towards your ears. Exhale and relax your shoulders. Repeat for 5-10 reps.

12. Seated Triceps Stretch: Begin in the Seated Mountain Pose. Reach your right arm up and behind your back. Use your left hand to gently press your right elbow towards your back. Hold for 5-10 breaths before releasing and repeating on the left side.

13. Seated Chest Expansion: Begin in the Seated Mountain Pose. Inhale and reach your arms out to the sides. Exhale and bring your arms back in front of your chest. Repeat for 5-10 reps.

14. Seated Neck Stretch: Begin in the Seated Mountain Pose. Interlace your fingers behind your head. Inhale and lift your elbows up towards the sky. Exhale and press your elbows back behind your head. Hold for 5-10 breaths.

15. Seated Eagle Pose: Begin in the Seated Mountain Pose. Cross your right arm over your left and bend your elbows. Reach your hands forward and clasp your fingers together. Hold for 5-10 breaths before releasing and repeating on the left side.

16. Seated Warrior I Pose: Begin in the Seated Mountain Pose. Inhale and reach your arms up to the sky. Exhale and reach your right arm to the back of the chair. Cross your left arm over your right and press your palms together. Hold for 5-10 breaths before returning to center and repeating on the left side.

17. Seated Warrior II Pose: Begin in the Seated Mountain Pose. Inhale and reach your arms up to the sky. Exhale and reach your right arm to the back of the chair. Place your left hand on the outside of your right arm and press your palms together. Hold for 5-10 breaths before returning to center and repeating on the left side.

18. Seated Triangle Pose: Begin in the Seated Mountain Pose. Inhale and reach your arms up to the sky. Exhale and reach your right arm to the back of the chair. Place your left hand on the outside of your right arm and twist your torso to the right. Hold for 5-10 breaths before returning to center and repeating on the left side.

19. Seated Side Plank: Begin in the Seated Mountain Pose. Place your right hand on the arm of the chair and your left hand on the seat. Lift your hips off the seat and hold for 5-10 breaths before returning to center and repeating on the left side.

20. Seated Corpse Pose: Begin in the Seated Mountain Pose. Inhale and reach your arms up to the sky. Exhale and reach your arms out to the sides. Close your eyes and relax into the chair. Stay here for 5-10 breaths.

Chapter 6. Breathing Techniques

Chair yoga for seniors is a great way for them to improve their overall fitness and well-being. One of the main components of chair yoga is breathing techniques. Proper breathing techniques can help seniors relax and improve their overall physical and mental health.

1. Abdominal Breathing: Start by sitting comfortably in a chair with your feet flat on the floor. Place one hand on your abdomen and the other on your chest. Inhale slowly and deeply, focusing on pushing your abdomen out as you breathe in. Exhale slowly, allowing your abdomen to relax.

2. Ujjayi Breath: Sit in a comfortable position and begin to take long, slow breaths. As you inhale, lightly constrict the back of your throat, creating a "haa" sound. Allow the breath to flow out smoothly and continuously.

3. Diaphragmatic Breathing: Start by sitting comfortably in a chair with your feet flat on the

floor. Place one hand on your abdomen and the other on your chest. Inhale slowly, focusing on pushing your abdomen out. As you exhale, contract your abdominal muscles and allow the air to flow out of your body.

4. Alternate Nostril Breathing: Begin by sitting in a comfortable position and press your right thumb lightly against your right nostril. Inhale slowly through the left nostril and exhale through the right. Repeat the same process on the opposite side by pressing your left thumb against the left nostril and inhaling through the right.

5. Nadi Shodhana: Begin by sitting in a comfortable position and using your right hand, press your index and middle finger gently against the middle of your forehead. Close off your right nostril with your thumb and inhale slowly and deeply through the left nostril. Then switch and close off the left nostril with your ring and little finger and exhale through the right.

6. Four-Part Breath: Begin by sitting in a comfortable position, with your feet flat on the floor. Inhale deeply and slowly through your nose,

focusing on filling your abdomen, rib cage, and chest with air. Exhale slowly and deeply, allowing the air to move out of your body in the opposite order.

7. Bumblebee Breath: Begin by sitting in a comfortable position and take a few deep and slow breaths. Open your mouth slightly and start to make a humming sound, like a bumblebee, as you exhale. Continue this process for several breaths.

8. Sama Vritti: Begin by sitting in a comfortable position and take a few deep and slow breaths. Then inhale for a count of four, hold your breath for a count of four, and exhale for a count of four.

9. Skull Shining Breath: Begin by sitting in a comfortable position and take a few deep and slow breaths. As you exhale, focus on pushing the air out of your body through the crown of your head, as if you were shining a light from the inside.

10. Lion's Breath: Begin by sitting in a comfortable position and take a few deep and slow breaths. Then open your mouth as wide as you can, stick out your tongue and, as you exhale, make a "haaa" sound.

11. Ocean Breath: Begin by sitting in a comfortable position and take a few deep and slow breaths. As you inhale, make a long, low "ooh" sound and as you exhale, make a long, low "ahh" sound.

12. Bellows Breath: Begin by sitting in a comfortable position and take a few deep and slow breaths. Quickly inhale and exhale, making a "whoosh" sound with each breath.

13. Seated Cat/Cow Pose: Begin by sitting in a comfortable position and take a few deep and slow breaths. As you inhale, arch your back and tilt your head up. As you exhale, round your back and tilt your head down.

14. Alternate Breathing: Begin by sitting in a comfortable position and take a few deep and slow breaths. As you inhale, focus on breathing in through one nostril and as you exhale, focus on breathing out of the other nostril.

15. Cooling Breath: Begin by sitting in a comfortable position and take a few deep and slow breaths. Curl your tongue up and out, like a straw,

and then exhale through the straw-shaped hole in your tongue, making a hissing sound.

16. Humming Bee Breath: Begin by sitting in a comfortable position and take a few deep and slow breaths. Then inhale deeply, hold your breath and make a humming sound, like a bee, as you exhale.

17. Kapalabhati Breath: Begin by sitting in a comfortable position and take a few deep and slow breaths. As you exhale, use your abdominal muscles to push the air out of your body in short bursts.

18. Three-Part Breath: Begin by sitting in a comfortable position and take a few deep and slow breaths. Inhale slowly and deeply, filling your abdomen, rib cage, and chest with air. Hold the breath for a few seconds and then, as you exhale, focus on releasing the air from your body in three stages.

19. Bhramari Breath: Begin by sitting in a comfortable position and take a few deep and slow breaths. Then close your eyes, press your index fingers against your ears and make a low, humming sound, like a bee, as you exhale.

20. Victory Breath: Begin by sitting in a comfortable position and take a few deep and slow breaths. As you exhale, raise your arms above your head, spread your fingers wide and make a victory sound, like a "hoo-hah!".

Chapter 7. Cool Down Exercises

Cooling down exercises are an important part of any chair yoga session for seniors. These exercises help to reduce post-exercise heart rate, help to reduce lactic acid build-up, and help to reduce muscle soreness. Cool down exercises also help to gradually decrease body temperature, and help to reduce the risk of injury or strain.

Cooling down exercises can be done at the end of the yoga session, when the body is most relaxed. These exercises should be performed at a slow and smooth pace and should last for at least five minutes.

Cooling down exercises can include gentle stretches and range of motion exercises. These exercises should be done slowly and gently, without any jerking or bouncing movements. During these exercises, seniors should focus on their breathing and keeping their spine straight.

In addition to helping to reduce post-exercise heart rate and muscle soreness, cooling down exercises can also help to reduce stress levels and improve overall circulation. Cool down exercises can also help to reduce joint stiffness, improve flexibility, and improve overall balance.

1. Seated Cat-Cow: Begin seated with both feet flat on the floor and your hands on your knees. Inhale and arch your back, lifting your chest upward and allowing your gaze to lift upward. Exhale and round your spine, tucking your chin to your chest and drawing your navel in toward your spine. Continue for 5 breaths.

2. Seated Side Bends: Begin seated with both feet flat on the floor and your hands on your knees. Inhale and lift your right arm up and over to the left side of your body. Exhale and allow your right side to stretch and your right arm to move further overhead. Hold for 5 breaths and switch sides.

3. Seated Spinal Twist: Begin seated with both feet flat on the floor and your hands on your knees. Inhale and bring your right arm up and cross it over your body to the left side. As you exhale, twist your torso to the left and bring your right elbow to the

outside of your left knee. Hold for 5 breaths and switch sides.

4. Seated Knees to Chest: Begin seated with both feet flat on the floor and your hands on your knees. Inhale and draw your right knee up and in toward your chest. Wrap your arms around your knee and hold for 5 breaths. Release and switch sides.

5. Seated Ankle to Knee: Begin seated with both feet flat on the floor and your hands on your knees. Inhale and draw your right ankle up and in toward your left knee. Hold for 5 breaths and switch sides.

6. Seated Figure Four: Begin seated with both feet flat on the floor and your hands on your knees. Inhale and cross your right ankle over your left knee. Exhale and press your right knee away from you to deepen the stretch. Hold for 5 breaths and switch sides.

7. Seated Forward Fold: Begin seated with both feet flat on the floor and your hands on your knees. Inhale and reach your arms up and over your head. Exhale and hinge from your hips and fold forward. Allow your arms to dangle and hold for 5 breaths.

8. Seated Neck Rolls: Begin seated with both feet flat on the floor and your hands on your knees. Inhale and bring your chin up to your chest. Exhale and circle your head to the right. Inhale and continue to circle your head back to center. Exhale and circle your head to the left. Continue for 5 breaths.

9. Seated Shoulder Shrugs: Begin seated with both feet flat on the floor and your hands on your knees. Inhale and lift your shoulders up toward your ears. Exhale and shrug your shoulders away from your ears. Continue for 5 breaths.

10. Seated Hand Clasp: Begin seated with both feet flat on the floor and your hands on your knees. Inhale and reach your right arm up and over your head. Exhale and clasp your left hand around your right wrist. Hold for 5 breaths and switch sides.

Chapter 8. Safety Considerations

Safety considerations are of utmost importance when practicing chair yoga for seniors. Proper instruction and precautions must be taken to ensure a safe and enjoyable experience.

1. Check the environment for any obstacles that might interfere with the practice, such as furniture, pets, or toys.

2. Wear comfortable, non-binding clothing and supportive shoes.

3. Place a yoga mat or towel on the floor for traction and padding.

4. Adjust the chair to a comfortable height, with the back and arms supported.

5. Begin the practice slowly and avoid any sudden movements.

6. Focus on proper breathing to support the poses.

7. Listen to the body and move within a range of motion that feels comfortable.

8. Avoid any poses that cause pain or discomfort.

9. Drink plenty of water before, during, and after the practice.

10. If pain or dizziness occur, stop the practice and seek medical advice if needed.

11. Avoid deep forward bends and backbends.

12. Do not hold a pose for too long.

13. Do not strain the neck or shoulders.

14. Avoid any poses that require balancing on one foot.

15. Take breaks and rest when needed.

16. Stay hydrated during the practice.

17. Use props to support the body and increase comfort.

18. Avoid strenuous poses and focus on gentle stretching.

19. Be aware of any medical conditions that may impact the practice.

20. Practice with a friend or caregiver if possible.

Chapter 9. Tips For Incorporating Chair Yoga Into Daily Routine

Incorporating chair yoga into a daily routine for seniors is important for many reasons. Chair yoga is an accessible form of exercise for those with physical limitations or those who are unable to stand for long periods of time.

This type of yoga is also beneficial for seniors who are looking to improve their flexibility, balance, and strength. It is also a great way for seniors to relax and reduce stress, which in turn can improve their overall mental health.

Here are few tip;

1. Begin each day with a few chair yoga poses. Doing this will help you to wake up and prepare for the day.

2. Make sure to sit in a comfortable chair with your feet flat on the floor and your hands resting on your lap.

3. Take a few deep breaths to help relax your body and clear your mind.

4. Start with a few simple chair poses such as Seated Cat/Cow, Seated Twist, Seated Mountain, Seated Forward Fold and Seated Side Bend.

5. Hold each pose for at least five deep breaths.

6. Move slowly and mindfully through each pose.

7. Focus on your breathing and try to relax your body and mind.

8. Incorporate arm stretches into your routine. These can be done in a seated position, such as raising your arms above your head and reaching for the ceiling.

9. To increase the intensity of your poses, try adding light weights or resistance bands to your routine.

10. Try to do at least ten minutes of chair yoga each day.

11. Place your chair in front of a window or outdoors in nature to help increase the calming benefits of chair yoga.

12. If you have access to a yoga mat, place it underneath the chair for extra support.

13. Once you become more comfortable with chair yoga, you can try more advanced poses such as Chair Downward Dog, Chair Warrior I and Chair Warrior II.

14. Listen to calming music or a guided meditation to help you stay focused and relaxed.

15. Take breaks whenever you need them.

16. Incorporate yoga breathing exercises into your routine. For example, try inhaling for four counts and exhaling for eight counts.

17. Try to practice chair yoga at the same time each day to help make it part of your daily routine.

18. Incorporate chair yoga into your day by doing it while watching TV or talking on the phone.

19. Join an online yoga class or watch tutorial videos to help you learn new poses and techniques.

20. Lastly, remember to be gentle and kind to yourself. Chair yoga should be a relaxing experience.

Conclusion

The book "Chair Yoga for Seniors" has presented a full explanation of the benefits of yoga for seniors, in addition to providing a number of chair yoga postures and sequences that can enhance both one's physical and emotional wellbeing.

It is possible for seniors and those with limited mobility to benefit from a kind of exercise known as chair yoga, which allows participants to reap the therapeutic effects of yoga without having to get out of a chair or get up at any point during the practice.

The author of this book offers senior citizens the information and advice they need to enjoy the benefits of chair yoga in the comfort of their own homes and gracefully age.